# TABLE OF CONTENTS

# Shakes for Weight Loss

## Sassy Classy Strawberry Shake

Serves: 1

One SERVING: 297 calories, 24.3g protein, 6.3g fat, 36.4g carbs, 6.7g fiber

- 2 scoops (or 1 packet) IsaLean® Shake Natural Creamy Vanilla
- 1 scoop (or 1 packet) IsaFruits®
- 8 oz water
- Handful of ice
- ½ cup fresh strawberries
- 1 strawberry for garnish

Place all ingredients in an Blender and blend until creamy. Garnish with a fresh strawberry.

# Shakes for Weight Loss

## Lean Chai Express

- 2 scoops Vanilla IsaLean Shake
- 8 ounces purified water
- 1 handful ice
- 1 1/2 cups chilled brewed chai tea
- 1/2 banana (only 40 calories!)
- 1/2 teaspoon cinnamon
- Optional (1 teaspoon honey)

Blend and enjoy!

# Shakes for Weight Loss

## Strawberry Slimmer

- 2 scoops Vanilla IsaLean Shake
- 8 ounces purified water
- 1 handful ice
- 1 scoop IsaFruits
- 1/2 cup strawberries (only 25 calories!)
- 1/2 teaspoon vanilla extract

Blend and enjoy!

# Shakes for Weight Loss

## Harvest Apple Pie Shake

- 2 scoops Natural Creamy Vanilla IsaLean® Shake
- 8 oz water
- Ice
- 1 whole organic apple (cored, not peeled)
- Dash or two of cinnamon

Mix all ingredients in a Blender and enjoy!

# Shakes for Weight Loss

## Cherry Chocolate Shake

- 2 scoops IsaLean® Shake in Rich Chocolate
- 8 oz purified water
- Ice cubes (desired amount)
- 6 organic cherries

Blend well and serve cold.

# Shakes for Weight Loss

## Cookies 'N Cream Shake

- 8 oz. water and crushed ice
- 2 scoops IsaLean® Shake in Natural Creamy Vanilla
- 1/4 SlimCakes® in Oatmeal Berry

Blend ingredients together and enjoy!

# Shakes for Weight Loss

## Orange Energizer

- 2 scoops IsaLean® Shake in Natural Creamy Vanilla
- 1 Tbsp Want More Energy?® in Orange
- 1 scoop Isagenix FiberPro™
- 8 oz Water and ice

Mix all ingredients in Blender and serve cold.
Enjoy!

# Shakes for Weight Loss

## Peppermint Patty Shake

- 8 oz crushed ice and water
- 2 Scoops IsaLean® Shake in Natural Creamy Chocolate
- 1/2 tsp vanilla extract, 1/2 tsp peppermint extract

Blend in Blender and enjoy!

# Shakes for Weight Loss

## Piña Colada Shake

- 2 scoops IsaLean® Shake in French Vanilla
- ¼ cup fresh or frozen pineapple
- ¼ teaspoon coconut extract
- 8 oz purified water

Blend well and serve cold.

# Shakes for Weight Loss

## Shamrock Shake

- 2 scoops IsaLean® Shake in Natural Creamy Vanilla
- 8 oz purified water
- ¼ teaspoon IsaFruits®
- 1 scoop Isagenix Greens!™
- 1 handful of ice

Blend until creamy and serve.

# Shakes for Weight Loss

## Milk Chocolate Peanut Butter Cups

- 1 scoop IsaLean® Shake in Natural Creamy Chocolate
- 1 scoop IsaLean® Shake in Natural Creamy Vanilla
- 1 square IsaDelight Plus™ Milk or Dark Chocolate
- 1 tsp. Natural Peanut Butter
- 8 oz. of water

Blend with ice

# Shakes for Weight Loss

## Hawaiian Hibiscus

- 2 scoops IsaLean® Shake in Natural Creamy Chocolate, Natural Creamy Vanilla or one scoop of each
- 1/2 to 1 scoop IsaCalcium®
- 2 scoops Tropical Fruit & Hibiscus Want More Energy?®
- 8 oz. of water

Blend with ice

# Shakes for Weight Loss

## Blueberry

- 1/2 cup washed organic blueberries
- 1 scoop Isagenix FiberPro™
- 1 scoop IsaCalcium®
- 8 oz. of water

Blend with ice

# Shakes for Weight Loss

## Mango Madness

- 2 scoops IsaLean® Shake in Natural Creamy Vanilla
- 1/2 scoop Orange Want More Energy?®
- 1/4 to 1/2 cup frozen or fresh Mangos
- 8 oz. of water

Blend with ice

Garnish with a slice of orange or Mango

# Low-Cal Entrees

## Tasty-Healthy-Chili

### Serves: 4 people

- 2 packets Savory Tomato IsaLean® Soup
- 3 1/4 cup water
- 2 bell peppers, diced (yellow, red)
- 1 tsp red pepper flakes
- 3 tsp black pepper
- 1 tsp garlic powder
- 1 lb ground turkey
- 1 can organic black beans

**Directions:**

Put water and peppers in a pot and bring to a boil.

Coat pan with olive oil cooking spray. Season turkey to your liking and fry until completely cooked (you can even add onions).

Add 2 IsaLean packets, turkey, seasonings and beans to water.

Reduce heat to low.

Let simmer for roughly 10-15 minutes, stirring often, until done.

# Low-Cal Entrees

## Carrot Apple Crunch Roll Ups

Serves: 1

One serving: 420 calories, 14.4g protein, 14.4g fat, 58.6g carbs, 5.0g fiber

- 1 sprouted-wheat tortilla*
- ¼ cup low-fat hummus*
- 2 tsp IsaCrunch® (hulled hemp seeds)
- ¼ cup julienned carrots
- ½ red apple, sliced
- ½ cup arugula leaves

Warm the tortilla, so it's pliable. Spread the hummus over the tortilla. Sprinkle IsaCrunch on the hummus. Layer with carrots, apples, and arugula. Roll tightly together and refrigerate.

*Nutrition info may change based on actual tortilla and hummus used.

# Low-Cal Entrees

## Encrusted Salmon Crunch

Serves: 2

One SERVING: 190 calories, 9.2g fat, 24.7g protein, 0.8g carbs, 0.2g fiber

- 1 tsp olive oil
- 2, 4oz filets of salmon
- 3 tsp IsaCrunch® hulled hemp seeds
- Pinch of cinnamon
- ¼ tsp salt
- Dash of pepper

Brush filets with olive oil. Mix IsaCrunch, cinnamon, salt and pepper in a small bowl. Sprinkle or press mixture onto salmon filets. Bake or broil (mixture side up) to desired temperature or when fish begins to flake.

Serving suggestion: Enjoy with a side of your favorite vegetable.

# Low-Cal Entrees

## Chicken Soup with Brown Rice

Serves: 1

One SERVING: 445 calories, 24.5g protein, 7.1g fat, 69.0g carbs, 6.5g fiber

- 1 serving (or 1 packet)
- IsaLean® Soup Classic Creamy Chicken
- 8 oz water
- 1 tbsp pine nuts
- 1 cup cooked (¼ cup uncooked) brown rice
- ½ medium tomato, diced
- 2 tsp fresh basil, finely chopped
- 2 tsp fresh parsley, finely chopped
- ¼ tsp salt
- Dash of pepper

Make one serving IsaLean Soup Classic Creamy Chicken. In a separate pot, make brown rice. Ten minutes before brown rice finishes cooking, stir in pine nuts, tomato, basil, parsley, salt and pepper. Before serving, add rice medley to soup.

# Low-Cal Entrees

## Cucumber Cashew Roll

- 1 tortilla
- 3 teaspoons IsaCrunch® premium hulled hemp seeds
- ½ cup chopped cucumber
- 1 cup chopped romaine lettuce
- ½ medium-size tomato – chopped
- 6 raw cashews—chopped

**Olivella Dressing (for Cucumber Cashew Roll)**

- 1 tablespoon olive oil
- 1 tablespoon lemon juice
- 1 teaspoon white vinegar
- ½ teaspoon fresh parsley—finely chopped
- 1 medium clove garlic—minced
- Salt/pepper to taste

Warm the tortilla, then brush with a very light coat of the Olivella Dressing. Sprinkle IsaCrunch atop tortilla. Mix together your lettuce, cucumber, cashews and tomato. Drizzle with remaining dressing and toss lightly. Place mixture evenly atop tortilla. Roll tightly and enjoy.

# Low-Cal Entrees

## Protein Pancakes

Makes 6 pancakes

Per 2 pancakes - Calories: 275, Fat 14 g, Carbs 25 g, Protein 25 g

- 6 egg whites beaten until fluffy
- 1/2 cup uncooked old fashioned oats
- 1/2 cup of fat free cottage cheese
- 1/2 scoop IsaLean Vanilla
- 1/2 scoop IsaPro
- ¼ cup IsaCrunch
- ¼ cup wheat germ
- 1 teaspoon baking powder
- 1 tablespoon canola oil
- ½ tsp cinnamon

Optional ingredients – 4 IsaDelight Plus chopped, ½ cup blueberries or 1 scoop IsaFruits

**Directions:**

Place all ingredients into blender except egg whites. Pulse until mixture is uniform. Pour into bowl and fold in egg whites. Heat griddle, cook and serve.

## Spinach & Strawberry IsaCrunch Salad

Number of Servings: 8

Per Serving - Calories 235, Total Fat: 15 g

- 2 bunches spinach, rinsed and torn into bite-size pieces
- 4 cups sliced strawberries
- 1/2 cup IsaCrunch
- 1/2 cup vegetable oil
- 1/4 cup white wine vinegar
- 1/4 cup sugar
- 1/4 teaspoon paprika
- 2 tablespoons sesame seeds
- 1 tablespoon poppy seeds

**Directions:**

In a large bowl, toss together the spinach and strawberries.

In a medium bowl, whisk together the oil, vinegar, sugar, paprika, sesame seeds, and poppy seeds. Pour over the spinach and strawberries along with the IsaCrunch® and toss to coat.

# Low-Cal Entrees

## Baked Chicken Nuggets

Number of servings: 6 – 4 nuggets per serving

- 3 boneless, skinless chicken breasts weighing about 6 oz. each
- 1/4 cup of oat bran
- 1/4 cup of IsaCrunch
- 1/4 cup coarsely ground almonds
- 1/2 teaspoon sea salt
- 1/2 teaspoon white pepper
- Pinch garlic powder
- 1/2 cup water or low-sodium chicken broth
- 1 large egg white, lightly beaten

**Directions:**

Preheat oven to 400°F. Prepare baking sheet by lining with parchment paper or coating lightly with best-quality olive oil.

Cut chicken breasts into nugget-sized pieces, about 1.5 inches square. Set aside. Next, combine all dry ingredients in a large container with a tightly fitting lid. Shake well. This is your coating mixture.

Combine water and egg in a medium bowl. Dip each piece in the water/egg-white mixture. Then dip each piece in the coating mixture. Make sure each piece is well coated.

Place on the baking sheet. When all of your chicken has been coated and your baking sheet is full, place in the oven and bake for 10-15 minutes or until golden.

# Low-Cal Entrees

## Cold Poached Salmon with Ginger

Yields: 4 servings

Calories: 375 per serving

- 4 salmon steaks
- 1/2 cup dry white wine
- 1 bay leaf
- 4-5 peppercorns
- 1/2 cup plain nonfat yogurt
- 2 tablespoons brown sugar
- 2 tablespoons nonfat mayo
- 2 tablespoons green onions finely chopped
- 2 teaspoons ginger

**Directions:**

In large skillet combine wine, water, bay leaf, and peppercorns

Heat to boil

Add salmon and cover

Simmer 5-7 minutes turning once

Transfer to plate and refrigerate for 2 hours *(Continued on next page)*

In a small bowl, combine yogurt, mayo, and green onions.
Spoon ginger over fish

**Side Dish Suggestions:**

1/2 cup of brown rice
Steamed vegetables of choice
Steamed carrots or baby yellow squash

# Low-Cal Entrees

## Spicy Chicken Soup

Yields: 2 servings

Calories: 400-500 per serving

- 4 scoops IsaLean® Soup in Classic Creamy Chicken
- 16 oz purified water, cold
- ¼ cup organic broccoli, chopped
- ¼ cup organic corn, cooked or raw off of the cob
- Pepper to taste
- ¼ cup green salsa
- Jalapeno peppers (to taste) finely diced
- 1 tablespoon IsaCrunch™
- Organic chicken pieces or assorted steamed vegetables (optional)

**Directions:**

Place broccoli and corn in a pan on low heat or in a steamer

Add black pepper and fresh garlic

In IsaBlender™, mix soup with cold water

Add green salsa and jalapenos

Blend together and add to veggies over low heat

Add organic chicken pieces or assorted steamed vegetables (optional)

Sprinkle IsaCrunch™ on top and serve.

# Low-Cal Entrees

## Hummus Sandwich

Yields: 1 serving

Calories: 400-500

- 3 tablespoons hummus
- 1 slice tomato
- 2 slices whole wheat or healthy bread

# Low-Cal Entrees

## Ginger-Curry Soup

Yields: 2 servings
Calories: 400-500 per serving

- 4 scoops IsaLean® Soup in Classic Creamy Chicken
- 16 oz purified water, cold
- 1 teaspoon spicy yellow curry powder
- Pinch of organic ginger (fresh or powdered)
- 1 cup organic brown rice, already cooked
- 1 medium organic yellow potato, cooked and diced
- Leafy green vegetables of your choice, chopped into medium-sized pieces

**Directions:**

Blend the first four ingredients well

Cook over low heat (do not boil or the enzymes could be

compromised). Cooks quickly so watch closely.

Add rice, potatoes and veggies.

# Low-Cal Entrees

## Oriental Salad

Yields: 1 serving

Calories: 450 per serving

- 1/2 cup each shredded Bibb lettuce and fresh spinach leaves
- Almond shavings (use sparingly)
- 1/4 cup drained mandarin oranges
- 1/4 cup herbed croutons
- 2 tablespoons each white vinegar and olive oil

**Directions:**

Mix lettuce, spinach and oranges.

Toss with white vinegar and olive oil

Sprinkle lightly with almond shavings and herbed croutons.

# Low-Cal Entrees

## Chicken in Orange Sauce

- 4 - 4 oz chicken breasts (or turkey)
- 1/2 teaspoon paprika
- 1 medium onion sliced
- 1/2 cup frozen orange juice concentrate
- 2 tablespoons brown sugar
- 1 teaspoon soy sauce, low sodium
- ½ teaspoon ground ginger
- 4 teaspoon sherry

**Directions:**

Brown chicken pieces under broiler *(Continued on next page)*

Place in a Pam-coated casserole dish

Sprinkle with paprika

Arrange onion slices over chicken

Combine juice concentrate, brown sugar, parsley, soy sauce, ginger, water, and sherry. Pour over chicken and onions.

Cover and simmer until chicken is tender (approx. 35-45 min).

## Side Dish Suggestions:

1/2 cup brown rice

Steamed carrots with raisins

Steamed green beans

# Low-Cal Entrees

## Snapper and Salsa

Yields: 4 servings

Calories: 450 per serving

- 1 ½ pounds snapper
- 1/4 cup cilantro minced
- 1/2 yellow and green peppers, seeded and minced
- 1 small sweet onion, minced
- 1 cup pineapple, minced
- 1 tablespoon olive oil
- Juice of 2 limes

**Directions:**

Mix cilantro, peppers, onions and pineapple

Cover and chill

Combine oil and fresh lime juice

Spray vegetable oil on grill or pan and cook snapper for approximately 4-8 minutes on each side, basting occasionally with the lime juice mixture

Top with salsa and serve

**Side Dish Suggestions:**

1/2 cup brown rice

Cucumber wedges

# Low-Cal Entrees

## Very Veggie Salad

Yields: 1 serving
Calories: 400

- 1 cup spinach and/or lettuce
- 2 cup favorite vegetables
- 1/4 cup beans (red, garbanzos)
- 2 tablespoons balsamic vinegar
- 1 tablespoon olive oil

**Directions:**

Mix vegetables

Toss lightly with balsamic vinegar and olive oil

# Low-Cal Entrees

## Grilled Chicken Breast Salad

Yields: 1 serving

Calories: 400

- 1 cup lettuce
- 1 grilled chicken breast
- 1/4 cup croutons
- 1 tablespoon grated parmesan cheese

**Directions:**

Mix lettuce, chicken and parmesan cheese

Toss lightly with dressing

Top with croutons

# Low-Cal Entrees

## Beef and Spinach Stir Fry

Yields: 1 serving
Calories: 250

- 4 oz steak of choice
- 1/4 cup boiling water
- 1 tablespoon beef bouillon granules
- 1 tablespoon low sodium soy sauce
- 1/2 teaspoon sugar
- 1/2 teaspoon grated fresh ginger root
- Pinch crushed red pepper
- 1 medium carrot shredded
- 1 green onion in 1 inch pieces
- 1/4 pounds fresh spinach leaves, chopped

## Directions:

Trim excess fat from steak. Slice across grain and set aside

Combine water and bouillon, and stir well. Add soy sauce, sugar, ginger root, and red pepper. Stir well and set aside.

*(Continued on next page)*

Coat skillet with cooking spray, heat to medium heat for 2 minutes

Add carrots and green onions, stir for 2 minutes

Remove from pan and set aside

Add steak to pan; stir fry 4 minutes. Add soy sauce mix

Bring to boil

Cover, reduce heat and simmer 4 minutes

Add vegetables and spinach to pan

Stir-fry 1 minute or until spinach wilts

Serve over 1/4 cup of hot cooked rice without salt

# Healthy Snacks

## No Bake Orange Creamsicle Protein Bars

Yields: 9 bars

- Nonstick extra virgin olive oil cooking spray
- 1 1/2 cups dry old fashioned oats
- 3 scoops Vanilla IsaPro®
- 1 stick Orange Want More Energy?®
- 2 Tbsp IsaCrunch® or flaxseeds
- 1 cup nonfat dry powdered milk
- 1/4 cup natural peanut butter
- 1/2 cup warm water
- 1 tsp vanilla extra

## Directions:

Spray an 8 x 8 inch square baking pan with nonstick cooking spray; set pan aside

In a large bowl, combine oats, Vanilla IsaPro, Orange Want More Energy?, IsaCrunch or flaxseeds and nonfat dry powdered milk.

*(Continued on next page)*

In a separate bowl, whisk together peanut butter, water and vanilla.

Add peanut butter mixture to dry ingredients and mix until dough is sticky.

Using wet hands or a rubber spatula sprayed with nonstick cooking spray, and spread the mixture evenly into a 8 x 8 sprayed pan.

Freeze for 1 hour until mixture is firm enough to cut.

Cut into 9 squares.

Wrap individually and store in refrigerator or freezer until hungry.

# Healthy Snacks

## Tomato Garden Salsa

Serves: 4

One serving: 36 calories, 1.3g protein, 0.4g fat, 7.9g carbs, 1.8g fiber

- 2-3 medium-sized fresh tomatoes (from 1 lb to 1 ½ lbs), stems removed, finely diced
- 1 jalapeño chili pepper* (stems, ribs, seeds removed), finely diced
- 1 Serrano chili pepper* (stems, ribs, seeds removed), finely diced
- ½ red onion, finely diced
- ½ cup chopped cilantro
- Juice of one lime
- 1 tbsp Isagenix Greens!™

- Salt and pepper to taste
- Optional: oregano and/or cumin to taste

**Directions:**

Combine all of the ingredients in a medium-sized bowl and taste. If the chilies make the salsa too hot, add some more chopped tomato. If not hot enough, carefully add a few of the seeds from the chilies you set aside. Serve with cut up vegetables.

*Wash your hands thoroughly with soap and hot water after handling and avoid touching your eyes.*

# Healthy Snacks

## Sweet Dreamsicle

Serves: 6
One popsicle: 93 calories, 7.1g protein, 1.2g

fat, 11.3g carbs, 1.0g fiber

- 2 scoops (or 1 packet)
- IsaLean® Shake Natural Creamy Vanilla
- 2 tbsp IsaPro®
- 2 tbsp IsaFruits®
- 2 tbsp Want More Energy!® Orange

- 8 oz water
- Handful of ice
- 6 Popsicle stick molds with accompanying sticks

Place all ingredients in a Blender and blend until creamy.

Pour into Popsicle molds and freeze, adding sticks about halfway through freezing.

# Healthy Snacks

## Chocolate Crunch Custard

Serves: 2

One SERVING: 231 calories, 13.9g protein, 8.2g fat, 31.7g carbs, 7.5g fiber

- 2 scoops (or 1 packet) IsaLean® Shake Natural Creamy Chocolate
- 4 oz water
- Handful of ice
- 2 IsaDelight Plus™, chopped into small pieces

- 1 SlimCakes®, crumbled
- ½ cup fresh raspberries

Blend shake with water and ice in a Blender until creamy.

Pour mixture into bowl.

Add and stir in IsaDelight Plus.

Top with SlimCakes and fresh raspberries.

# Healthy Snacks

## Easy Bake Protein Bars

Number of Servings: 12
Per Serving — Calories 118, Fat 7 g, Carbs 18 g, Protein 15 g

- 3 cups uncooked old fashion oats
- 3 tablespoons milk powder, non-fat, dry organic
- 1 cup purified water
- 2 scoops IsaLean® Shake Vanilla

- 2 scoops IsaPro®
- 5 IsaDelight Plus™, chopped into small pieces
- 8 tablespoons unsalted natural peanut butter
- 2 packages stevia or other sweetener
- 2 teapoons IsaCrunch®

Mix all ingredients except IsaCrunch until well combined. Press into a 9 x 13 parchment-lined baking dish with wet hands.

Press IsaCrunch into the top and bake in a preheated, 350 degree oven for 20 minutes.

Let cool and cut into 12 squares.

# Healthy Snacks

## Frozen Protein Creamsicles

Number of Servings: 10
Per Serving — Calories 95, Fat <1 g, Carbs 14 g, Protein 8 g

- 2 cups fat-free Greek vanilla yogurt
- 1 scoop IsaLean Vanilla Shake
- 1 scoop IsaPro
- 1/2 cup purified water

- 2 scoops IsaFruits® or Isagenix Greens!™
- 6 ounces frozen orange juice concentrate
- 1 teaspoon of vanilla extract for added flavor
- Add 3 scoops of Want More Energy?® Orange for an extra boost!

Put all ingredients into a blender.

Blend until smooth.

Pour into individual molds, insert popsicle sticks and freeze.

# Tasty Drinks

## Sweet 'N Speedy Recovery Booster

- 12 ounces room temperature water
- 1 scoop IsaPro® Vanilla

- 2 scoops or ½ of 1 Stick of Want More Energy?® Tropical Fruit & Hibiscus
- Desired amount of ice (optional)

Fill your IsaShaker™ bottle with 12 ounces of room temperature, purified water

Add 1 scoop of IsaPro Vanilla and 2 scoops or ½ Stick of Want More Energy? Tropical Fruit & Hibiscus

Shake it up (burn a few extra calories while you're at it!)

Add your desired amount of ice and enjoy!

# Tasty Drinks

## Energizing Elixir

- 1 scoop Mars Venus Super Cleanse™

- 1 teaspoon Want More Energy?® in Citrus
- ¼ scoop Isagenix Greens!™
- 1 scoop IsaFruits®
- 8 oz purified water
- 10-12 ice cubes (for super-thick, slushy effect)

Blend well and serve.

# Tasty Drinks

## Warming Lemon Cleanse

- 1 scoop Mars Venus Super Cleanse™
- 8 oz hot, purified water

**Directions:**

Pour hot water into a large cup

Allow water to cool slightly

Add Mars Venus Super Cleanse™ and stir briskly

# Tasty Drinks

## Cool Cleanse Sorbet

- 1 scoop Natural Rich Berry Cleanse for Life® powder
- 1/2 scoop of IsaFruits®
- 3 oz. of water

- 4 oz. crushed ice

Blend in A Blender until consistency reaches that of a creamy sorbet.

# Kid-Friendly Fun Recipes

## Cinna-Fruity Shake

- 1 scoop IsaLean® Shake in Natural Creamy Vanilla
- 1 scoop IsaLean® Shake in Natural Creamy Chocolate
- 1 scoop IsaFruits®
- 1 tsp Cinnamon
- One-quarter of a banana
- 8 oz Water and ice

Mix ingredients in a Blender and serve cold.

Enjoy!

# Kid-Friendly Fun Recipes

## Berry Blast Shake

- 8-10 oz organic orange juice
- ½ banana
- 1 cup frozen berry medley (strawberries, blueberries and raspberries)
- 1 scoop IsaFruits®
- 1 scoop Isagenix Greens!™

Blend and enjoy.

# Kid-Friendly Fun Recipes

# OJ Shake

- 8 - 10 oz organic orange juice
- 2 scoops IsaLean® Shake in French Vanilla

- 1 squeeze of organic honey
- Ice (desired amount)

Blend and enjoy.

# Kid-Friendly Fun Recipes

## Bubblegum Shake

- 1 scoop IsaPro®
- 1 scoop IsaLean® Shake in French Vanilla
- 1 generous scoop of IsaFruits®
- ½ cup fresh or frozen pineapple chunks (5-6 chunks)
- 1 tablespoon Want More Energy?® in Citrus

Blend and enjoy.

# Kid-Friendly Fun Recipes

## Peanut Butter and Banana Shake

- 8-10 oz purified water
- 2 scoops IsaLean® Shake in French Vanilla
- 1 scoop organic peanut butter
- ½ banana
- Ice (desired amount)

Blend and enjoy

# Kid-Friendly Fun Recipes

## Carrot Charisma Shake

- 2 scoops IsaLean® Shake in French Vanilla
- 8 oz purified water
- 1 scoop Isagenix FiberPro™
- 1 scoop IsaFruits®
- 1 teaspoon IsaCalcium®
- 1 small/medium-sized organic carrot cut into pieces

Blend and enjoy.

# Kid-Friendly Fun Recipes

## Pink Lemonade

- 8 oz purified water
- 1 scoop Want More Energy?® in Citrus
- 1 scoop IsaFruits®.

Combine ingredients and enjoy!

# Kid-Friendly Fun Recipes

# Twin Power
# Super Shake

- 8 oz unsweetened organic rice drink
- 2 scoops IsaLean® Shake in Rich Chocolate
- 1 scoop IsaPro®
- 1 scoop IsaFruits®
- ½ cup organic strawberries
- Ice (desired amount)

Blend and enjoy.

## Shakes for Maintenance

# Dark Chocolate Peanut Butter Cup Shake

- 2 scoops IsaLean® Shake in Natural Creamy Chocolate
- 1 tsp decaffeinated coffee crystals
- 1 tsp peanut butter
- 8 oz water

Blend with ice

Shakes for Maintenance

# Coconut Cherry Dream Cream

- 1 scoop IsaLean® Shake in Natural Creamy Vanilla
- 1/2 of a banana (fresh or frozen), cherries, strawberries (substitutions may vary to liking)
- 1/4 cup coconut milk
- 1 tsp Orange Want More Energy?®
- 1 tsp IsaCalcium®
- 1 Tbsp shredded coconut

Add desired amount of ice and blend in a Blender

## Shakes for Maintenance

# Rip Roarin' Protein Shake

- 1 1/2 scoops IsaLean® Shake in Natural Creamy Chocolate
- 1 scoop IsaPro®
- 1 teaspoons Almond Butter
- 4 ounces Almond Milk
- 4 ounces purified water
- 2 ice cubes

Blend with an a Blender and enjoy!

Can also be eaten with a spoon.

# Shakes for Maintenance

# Egg Nog Delight

- 2 scoops IsaLean® Shake in Natural Creamy Vanilla
- 1/2 of a Banana
- 1 teaspoon Nutmeg
- 1 teaspoon Cinnamon
- 4 ounces purified water
- 4 ounces crushed ice

Blend with an a Blender and enjoy!

# Shakes for Maintenance

# Heavenly French Vanilla Shake

- 8 oz purified water
- 1 ½ scoops IsaLean® Shake in French Vanilla
- ½ scoop of IsaPro®
- ¾ of one SlimCakes®
- 2 tablespoons IsaCrunch™
- ½ scoop Isagenix Greens!™
- ½ cup crushed ice

Blend well and serve.

# Shakes for Maintenance

## Blueberry Blizzard

- 8 oz purified water
- 5-7 ice cubes
- 2 scoops IsaLean® Shake in French Vanilla
- 1 scoop IsaFruits®
- 1 scoop Isagenix Greens!™
- 1 teaspoon IsaCalcium®
- 1 scoop Isagenix FiberPro™
- ¼ cup organic frozen blueberries

Blend until thick and creamy.

# Shakes for Maintenance

## Key Lime Pie Shake

- 8 oz crushed ice and water
- 2 scoops IsaLean® Shake in Natural Creamy Vanilla
- 1/2 Want More Energy? ® Stick in Citrus
- 1 sheet honey graham crackers

Blend and enjoy!

# Shakes for Maintenance

## Pumpkin Pie Shake

- 8 oz crushed ice and water
- 2 scoops IsaLean® Shake in Natural Creamy Vanilla
- 3- 3 1/2 scoops of natural pumpkin (canned, 100% pumpkin) 1/2 Tbsp pumpkin pie spice (nutmeg, cinnamon, ginger, all spice)

Blend and enjoy!

# Shakes for Maintenance

## Chocolate Almond Biscotti Shake

- 2 scoops IsaLean® Shake in Natural Creamy Chocolate
- 2 scoops Orange Want More Energy?®
- 1 tsp. sliced almonds
- 8 oz. of water
- Desired amount of ice

Blend and enjoy!

# Shakes for Maintenance

## Strawberry-Banana Shake

- 2 scoops IsaLean® Shake in Natural Creamy Vanilla
- 1 handful frozen strawberries
- 1/2 medium banana
- 3 oz. plain, low-fat yogurt
- 8 oz. of water
- Desired amount of ice

Add ingredients, blend and enjoy!

www.ingramcontent.com/pod-product-compliance
Lightning Source LLC
Chambersburg PA
CBHW080629030426
42336CB00018B/3136